Nature's N

The Everyday Guide to Herbal Remedies & Healing Recipes for Common Ailments

Elizabeth Fellow

Elizabeth Fellow

Table of Contents

Introduction

With prescription charges rocketing and evermore drug resistant bugs and germs raising their diseased little heads many people are searching for alternatives to the traditional doctor's medicine. But which herbs and plants are safe to use and how can you decipher remedies from urban myth? This book holds the answer.

Meander down the garden path to learn how to heal common complaints such as diarrhoea, headaches and eczema. Improve your sex life using simple flowers most of us have growing in our own back yards. Fight bugs and germs quickly with delicious recipes. Every set of ingredients has been chosen for its healing properties and great tasting potential. Heck, the few nasty shockers even come with warnings!

This fail safe book takes you from interested amateur to reassured healer in a few short pages. Simple to use, it comes in three concise sections.

First: dip in and congratulate yourself on the benefits of the contents of your fruit bowl and fridge.

Next: learn how to make syrups, macerations and tinctures. Explore the tools of the healer's box and discover easy ways to apply salves and poultices.

Finally, experiment with preventative medicine and treatments in delicious recipes. Wind your way through weird and wonderful recipes from Auntie Violet's Sleepy Syrup for insomnia to Baked Papaya and Ginger Soothing Hug to chase away those colds and sneezes.

So if you are ready to feel healthier, look better and even step away from aches and pains......

Turn the page!

The Origins of folk medicine

Whilst the 21st century would seem to herald the new dawn of a natural healing, in fact we can trace folk medicine right through the annals of time. In many ways we are simply going back to "the old ways." As far back as the ancient Egyptians we can find evidence of the use of plant extracts. In excavations of tombs in the Valley of the Kings there have been discoveries of small tears of frankincense and myrrh. Much later the Bible tells of the magi bringing the same precious extracts to a baby in a manger. Frankincense, more valuable than gold, and of course myrrh was for the embalming of kings. Never were there more symbolic gifts given at a birth.

The Ancient Egyptians

The Egyptians had begun to experiment with the use of plant essences way back in the 3rd century BC. These perfumes, herbs and spices were to become some of the most sought after commodities in international trade. Camels pulled massive caravans of fragrant and delicious seasonings across the deserts both for cookery but also for use in healing and prayer. Their commodities were a prized and treasured load.

They understood how the plants separated themselves from their essences and played with ways to make the magic happen. During Cleopatra's reign (around 40 years before the birth of Christ) rose petals were strewn along the waters of the Nile in preparation for the queen's procession down the river. As the oils evaporated a heady aroma led her people into blissful ecstasy of her beauty. Legend has it that the like of her beauty had never before been seen anywhere in the world. One wonders how much of the glory came from the magic of the essences of her blooms.

Spikenard and Galbanum, oils lesser known today, but they too are mentioned many times in Bible too and their references show is just how valuable and highly prized they were during those times. They are used as examples of the majesty of the temple of Solomon.

Pliny the Elder

In AD 77 Pliny the Elder, a famed and well-loved naturalist wrote his epic work Naturalis Historica. Subsequently many encyclopaedias have taken their botanical references from this journal. Throughout the work he alludes to the healing capabilities of many plants we know and recognise today. He regales the benefits of dock, nettles and rosehips to name but a few. He was an extremely prolific author but of all his works, Naturalis Historica is the only one to have survived his death during the eruption of Mount Vesuvius.

The Ancient Greeks

It is amazing to think of the clarity of knowledge about plant medicine in the ancient world. When we look at Roman texts we see that they were developing a very clear understanding about *how* to heal, even then. The most famous of their doctors was a man called Galen (AD 129-200). He was a visionary in medicine, well ahead of his time. He was criticised by contemporaries for his refusal to accept symptoms were simply attributed to mysticism or divination. He was recorded as having argued "we must wait and observe". Today this seems obvious to us. We are familiar with the route of diagnosis and prognosis, but the physicians of his day were not.

This recognition of how a disease can develop, morph and change was a ground breaking notion.

His work built a foundation for the work of Hippocrates in many aspects but Galen's most important contribution was in the exploration of the circulatory system. He was the first person to recognise the difference in colour between the darker venous blood and the lighter arterial blood.

He was an accomplished surgeon and in fact some of his theories about operations of the eye and the brain still hold true and are used today. He used plants extensively as salves to mend wounds. In fact Galen is attributed as having formulated Cold Cream.

Dioscorides

Another military doctor, this one working under Nero was Dioscorides. He was an avid collector and student of plants. Today, we still refer to his notes in the 5 volumes of the Materia Medica.

Hippocrates

Hippocrates is considered to be the father of medicine. He built on the works Galen had begun. He gave us the understanding that illness comes from something which is wrong within the body. From him too we get the Hippocratic Oath. In his writings he mentions a vast number of plants. Later the books were translated into Arabic and can now be found in the modern library of Alexandria.

Avicenna

At this point the studies into plants and their properties gained great interest in the Arab countries. The greatest of all the contributions came from a physician called Abu Ali Ibn Sina (980-1037 AD). In writings you may also see his name as Avicenna. He writes extensively about his adventures experimenting with plants for beauty and for tonics. We cannot be sure if he invented distillation but there are many pictures of stills in his work. It seems likely that rose oil was the first to be used and may have been uncovered purely by accident during some other alchemical endeavours.

The Dark Ages

As one would imagine, we have very little documentation pertaining to the Dark Ages. By the 12th Century however, we can see plants were being moved from continent to continent, as the Crusaders bought back treasures from their travels. Previously in Europe the like of aromatic gums and resins had never been seen, their parent trees only swaying in the warm breezes of much warmer climes. As the Europeans began to use herbal waters and oils, blends began to be formed from these new travellers.

Medieval Medicine

By the 15th century, although Apothecaries sold essential oils, most large houses had their own still room to make the most of the plants in their gardens. Many herbals were written, the greatest in 1653 by English botanist Nicholas Culpepper, who remains a household name today.

The Age Of Reason

Skip forward now to the 17th and 18th centuries. What we call "The Age Of Reason" was starting to take hold along with so-called logical thinking. "Plant medicine" was pushed back to allow for a whole new world of chemical substances.

Meanwhile one German physician plugged away regardless and through his lifetime Friedrich Hoffman produced much of the information we know today about plant medicine.

During the 18th and 19th centuries scientists made a huge leap forward in healing when they identified that within plants were active ingredients which were very useful in medicines. For example quinine, digitalis and morphine were all formulated. All of which we use today. They removed the active ingredient from the plant and only used the part which seemed to bring about the response they needed in the body. Later you will see why this particular moment is so important in holistic medicine.

20th Century Resurgence

Throughout the 20th century, slowly but surely the healing knowledge began to change. Radicals such as Dr Jean Valnet and Marguerite Maury refused to be quietened by the medical establishment and continued to laud and investigate the power of plants.

The 1960s saw a dramatic divergence in the healing arts when experimentation of drugs leaked over into the hallucinogenic qualities of plants. The esoteric movement started to make connections between the mind –body and spirit and how they may be linked together in wellness.

Every day now holistic medicine becomes more complicated and in turn more closely regulated. Today we not only rely on the essences, herbals and plants themselves for their physical effects but we link them together with a whole range of other tools to encourage healing. A good therapist will look at their patient holistically. That is…. as a *whole* person.

We understand the importance of good spinal alignment for health. We assess dietary needs and vitamin therapy. Acupressure, Chinese medicine and reflexology can be used to enhance the benefits of the oils for detoxification of the body. Most of all we consider the emotions with counselling and meditation techniques.

At the beginning of this century essential oils and herbal remedies were on the shelves of every pharmacy and even supermarket, but changes in UK trading laws in 2010 across meant that many of these were removed. Other countries quickly followed suit. Restrictions and labelling legislation dictate now that only qualified professionals are able to sell complementary medicines.

Our responsibility

In some ways too, this history only covers what we know from the written history of the "civilised" world. Western arrogance, of course, because it is estimated that in less developed countries over 50% of the world rely entirely on plant medicine. Their knowledge of healing through the earth's (and include in that ocean's, soils and gemstone) resources far outstrips any of the knowledge we have here. Perhaps we did once know it but now it has been forgotten.

Just as in every evolution there is good and bad, plant medicine has its own challenges and opportunities. The introduction of antibiotics, especially penicillin saved many thousands of lives and will continue to do so. Interestingly just as we happily accept that super-bugs evolve and develop resistance to the doctor's drugs, so too does nature evolve its medicine. Plant qualities change their structure to keep up with the medicinal needs of our planet. The solution which halted the epidemic of Tamiflu three years ago was found in the spice, star anise.

What happens though, when an active constituent is identified which could solve a massive planetary problem, but resources are limited? This is happening at this very moment, scientists suspect that a certain type of coral on the Great Barrier Reef may hold the key to treatment for pancreatic cancer. And yet how could there possibly be enough of such a precious ingredient to go around? Exactly this happened to the poor Chinese take-aways when in the Swine Flu epidemic, there were no star anise to be found for about 3 months because every bit of resource was being used to try and stem the fatal illness.

We know the results of such an imbalance of supply and demand; extinction. In many cases in the past the ways of collecting aphrodisiacs, hallucinogens, or healing products were at best irresponsible and a worst barbaric. Running out of star anise is not so frightening in the grand scheme of things, it is a fast grower. But measure it against the sandalwood tree, which with extensive deforestation in India (not only for medicine, but also its beautiful wood for furniture) has taken the plant close to extinction. It takes 60 years for a Sandalwood

Tree to grow into a usable resource. Now that really is a problem.

A great responsibility lies on our shoulders. We are being given a second chance to rediscover these natural gifts, but this time with the knowledge of what harm we can also do. We who understand the Earth's capability to provide must protect this resource for the future generations.

Just as I hope to be able to convey the medicine to you, I would love to think you will want to take up a small part of your own garden, or even some pots on the windowsill, and grow some of your own medicine. After all, that which we take, we really should replace.

This book will merely scratch the surface of how to use "the old ways" to heal, but hopefully may take just a small step to bridge the gap between the availability of these wonderful natural medicines and the knowledge needed to use them to their full potential. No longer, are these remedies considered quack medicine. You are the first of many generations of the new healers.

Just for fun (You already know more than you think)

Not all plant medicine is arcane; much of it is very much ensconced in our human psyches. Here are some very fundamental facts which I think you will recognise:

1. If nature offers a threat, she will usually give you an antidote with it close by. Where there are nettles, so there are dock leaves to ease the pain of the stingers.
2. At school you may have been told not to pick dandelions because they made you want to go to the

bathroom. Dandelions are diuretic (albeit not as strong as the saying may suggest).

3. Prunes and curries are laxative.
4. If you have a cold, lemon and honey is the way forward.
5. Oranges for a strong constitution.
6. Eat greasy lamb with digestive mint sauce or rosemary jelly to avoid indigestion.
7. Some mushrooms are hallucinogenic.

Ok, so let's move on. We have seen how folk medicine has developed and changed but what does natural medicine look like now?

Forms of Today's Healing Medicines

Legend would have us believe that the apothecarists and the healers of old were strange old people living in the woods; witches and warlocks, hidden deep in the darkness, sought out only when magic was needed. How true that is we can only guess.

What we do know is these healers were also the midwives, the doctors and in many cases the funeral directors too. The woods, of course are a fabulous place to forage and grow all manner of unusual (and possibly slightly suspect things too) perhaps the woodlands would be likely for some, but probably not all.

Today's healers are everywhere though. Find them in high rise flats, in board rooms and most of all simply out in the world, just doing their thing! Here are some of the tools of their trade.

Essential Oils and Aromatherapy

One of the biggest growth areas of the twenty first century must surely be aromatherapy. The concentrated essences of plants are now readily available and most of us are at least familiar with the relaxing effects of lavender and perhaps the antiseptic qualities of tea tree. But if you were interested to explore deeper into these sweet smelling bottles what could you expect to find?

You have heard the phrase if I could bottle that goodness I'd b a millionaire? Well, meet the essential oils business! The parts of the plant which heal are captured in a way that can be easily applied to the body.

How does aromatherapy work?

Our skin is porous, which is why we turn into prunes if we stay in the bath too long. The molecules of the oils are small enough to absorb through the skin and into the blood stream. This process called osmosis takes around 20 minutes to complete. Once in the circulatory system they can flush to the internal organs requiring physical healing.

Our bodies run almost entirely on hormones. They govern how well our organs work. Most of the regulation of these hormonal levels is done by an organ in the brain called the hypothalamus. Its stem runs down from the base of the brain and into the spinal cord and governs how our emotions affect our organs. (Think: experiencing diarrhoea when you are nervous.) Essential oils are extremely effective in instructing the hypothalamus to raise or lower certain hormone levels to make organs work better.

For the main part then, aromatherapy finds ways to get the oils through the skin. Common methods of application are massage, creams and lotions, and putting oils in the bath.

When heated, essential oil molecules evaporate into the atmosphere. As they travel up the nose they pass along the olfactory system and into the brain. Here they activate what is called the Limbic System, whose job it is to control learning, spatial awareness, memory and above all emotions. Again, this is another dimension to having oils in the bath, but essential oils can also be used in evaporators and diffusers.

The oils are made up of many different parts, alcohols, acids, terpenes, the list goes on and on. Scientists can determine how an oil may be able to heal by analysing its chemistry. One particularly important part, called a sesquiterpene, has been identified as one of the only chemicals which is able to cross the blood brain barrier. This means that plant essences may herald a new dawn for medicines for diseases such as Parkinson's disease or Lupus.

Since essential oils are so concentrated it is important they be diluted before use in some sort of carrier. Often this will be a vegetable oil such as sunflower, olive, rosehip or coconut. Each have their own properties which can improve a blend further, but it is safe and economical experiment with what is in your cupboard. The only warning I would give here, is many are made from nuts and kernels of fruits and so take extra care of using on anyone with a nut allergy.

Dilutions

Always think less is more when using aromatherapy. Oils are expensive and extremely potent. Using too heavy a blend makes no sense as the body simply excretes any surplus as waste. The general rule of thumb is to use one or two drops only of an oil at a time. Feel free to add more different oils to it though.

Use one drop of oil to 25 drops of carrier at the very minimum.

Herbals

Herbals can be found in your local natural health shop and online. The medicines controls act legislation in many countries forbids the manufactures to publish the healing properties of these tablets on their labelling therefore it is worth checking out good websites such as Mountainroseherbs.com to get a good understanding of which ones can help you most.

Familiar ones which you may already recognise are Evening Primrose oil for Premenstrual Tension, Borage (or Starflower) for menopausal symptoms and even Ginko Biloba from a bit more between-the-sheets action.

Herbals have the advantage over aromatherapy in that dosage is clearly written on the jar and they are easy to take in tablet form.

Seaweeds

In effect these are herbals too, but they are so rich in nutrients and healing properties they merit a few lines of their own.

Seaweed is the single best natural source of iodine which is fundamental to normal thyroid function. Interestingly, no land grown plants have a need for iodine so it does not present itself very readily in normal vegetable diets. Since the thyroid controls everything from our temperature and weight to our metabolism, seaweed a powerful tool to have at your disposal.

Kelp in particular is an excellent source of iron and zinc which means lustrous thick locks and far better immunity from bugs and germs.

Detoxifying very deeply, seaweed also makes a brilliant defence against cellulite. Flushing the toxicity out of the body means very quickly you can wave goodbye to that horrid orange peel looking skin on your thighs.

Clays

The sea gives us gifts in the form of seaweed and the land also has amazing healing properties hidden in its soils (gems too of course, but that's a different book!). Whilst eating soil is not generally your best plan, laid onto the skin clays can draw out impurities and condition the skin.

Vitamins and Minerals

Vitamin therapy is a book in its own right (well an entire library of books, in truth) but a quick overview will help you to see deeper into the alchemy of nature and how it has developed to feed, heal and nurture our bodies.

Vitamin A
Important for maintaining healthy skin, vitamin A also supports a normal respiratory tract and prevents coughs and colds etc.

Vitamin B
This vitamin breaks down into many, many subsections but on the whole it metabolises fats, prevents depression, aids concentration, and helps the body extract energy from its food.

Vitamin C
This aids tissue repair and wound healing and important for the immune system.

Vitamin D

Important to bones and skin, this vitamin does not come from food. This is only manufactured by our skin when it is exposed to sunlight. Many of us no longer produce enough vitamin D since we're covering up our skin and spending a far smaller portion of our time out in the fresh air.

Vitamin E

A powerful antioxidant, vitamin E supports nerves and bones. It also guards against cardio vascular disease.

Calcium

Important to bones and teeth, calcium also plays a major part in blood clotting, regulating heartbeat and healthy skin.

Copper

This is a trace element, but without it we cannot absorb iron from our food. It helps to form connective tissue, such as nerves and tendons and ensures good bone growth.

Iron

Boosting energy levels, iron is essential for transporting oxygen to every cell in the body.

Magnesium

Important for healthy bones and teeth and also muscle contraction, magnesium also regulates the heartbeat.

Phosphorous
This is essential to release the energy from proteins into the bodily cells.

Potassium
Regulating bodily fluids, potassium ensures correct functioning of the nerve impulses and maintains blood pressure.

Sodium
Controlling the electrolytes in the blood, sodium is essential for nerve and muscle function.

Sulphur
Often used in creams to treat eczema and acne, sulphur is an antifungal and antibacterial agent. It exists in every cell of our bodies.

Zinc
This looks after the reproductive system, fertility in particular. It regulates our sense of taste and also helps wounds to heal.

Natural Medicine in the Kitchen

How to make tinctures

Tinctures are popular ways to take herbal medicine because they have a very long shelf life and can be easily carried around in your pocket. Great, if you need to be taking your medicine frequently, tinctures preserve the plant matter in alcohol. Vodka is usually the liquor of choice but as long as it is tasteless and is more than 80% proof, the choice is yours.

Find a glass or ceramic container with a lid. Avoid metal as it reacts with the alcohol and changes the properties of the blend.

The ratio of herbs to alcohol varies dependant on whether they are dried or fresh.

Use as follows:

- Add enough fresh chopped herbs to fill the glass container. Cover with alcohol
    o OR
- Add 4 ounces (113g) of powdered herb with 1 pint (473ml) of alcohol (or vinegar/glycerine)
    o OR
- Add 7 ounces (198g) of dried herb material to 35 fluid ounces (1 liter) of alcohol (or vinegar/glycerine).

1. Stir herbs and alcohol with a blunt knife ensuring all air pockets are dispersed.
2. Seal the lid well and place in a dark, cool place for 2 weeks, shaking regularly.

3. When the time has elapsed, take a piece of muslin or a tea towel to catch all the plant matter and allow the liquid to seep through into a bowl below. Squeeze gently.
4. Decant the tincture into a small dark glass bottle and seal well. Label clearly and keep out reach of children.

Kept properly, a tincture has a shelf life of around five years.

How to make infusions

Infusions are remedies which are drunk, much like a cup of tea. 2 tablespoons of plant matter is placed in a jar, covered with boiling water and left to steep with a lid on, for between 4-6 hours.

How to make decoctions

Unlike infusions, decoctions use rigorous boiling as a means to extract the properties from more stubborn matter such as woods and spices.

Use a heavy pan and around 2 tablespoons of plant matter to 1 cup of water. Bring to a boil and then simmer for around 20 minutes.

Decant and allow to cool to drinking temperature before use.

How to make macerations

I mentioned carrier oils earlier, as a method to dilute essential oils. Many of these are macerations. In the summertime this is a wonderful way to capture the essences of the plants and create your own healing oils.

Fill a bottle or jar with the vegetable oil, any oil will do. Fill it full of plant matter, petals, herbs or spices and ensure they are completely covered with the oil. Leave it for a month on the windowsill in the sunshine. The vegetable oil takes the essential oils of the plant into it and you have a lovely magical oil. Rose petals for skin care, lemon balm to make massage oils to aid cognition in dementia patients and lavender oil to relax, these are all medicines you can make for pennies.

How to make a poultice

A poultice now may be called a compress. It is used to place herbs or oils onto the skin to either draw out toxin and poisons or to allow the herbs to sit atop a wound for quickest healing. Poultices can either be warm (to open the pores) or cold (to shut them down again). By alternating warm and cold, opening and closing the pores repeatedly, toxicity is drawn to the surface. This is useful in cases of abscesses or even nasty blemishes for example.

Soak a cloth in water, add the herbs and place over the wound. It can help to bandage the herbs in place. To add essential oils, add 3 drops to the water before soaking. Try to use extreme temperatures which are still comfortable, so the hottest or coldest you can bear. Always test the water for temperature to avoid scalding.

How to make inhalants

On the days when you have a cold and can hardly speak for being so stuffed up, this is your heaven sent solution.

Fill a large bowl with boiling water. Add herbs or oils and allow them to release their vapour into the steam. Put your face into the steam (not close enough to scald) and cover your head and to sides of the bowl with a large bath towel to trap the steam. Very quickly you will start to sweat and release the toxins in your skin. The vapours cut through the mucous build up in the sinuses. One warning…have your tissues at the ready and expect your nose to run!

Inhalants also make up an important part of skin care, allowing the skin to clean far more deeply than any other cleansing method.

5 – 10 minutes over an inhalation is plenty and always apply a moisturiser afterwards to replace all the hydration you have drawn away.

How to make syrups

Often tinctures and decoctions can be unpalatable to children. A syrup is the answer as it is sweet and comforting. Since the ratios of ingredients vary a great deal, I shall list them individually in the remedies section, but in each case the preparation is as follows.

1. Warm the fruit or herb until all its juices have been released into the water.
2. Gently add the sugar, bring to the boil and simmer for 10-15 minutes.
3. To test consistency, drip a droplet of the syrup into a glass of cold water. If it splits into pieces, boil a little longer.

If the drop remains intact, the syrup is ready to bottle into a sterilized container.

How to sterilize jars and bottles

Use only glass containers for herbal medicines. Wash with warm soapy water and rinse well. Do not towel dry. Place face down onto the rack shelves of a preheated oven at 150 degrees Fahrenheit /65 degrees Celsius and leave for 20 minutes.

Meanwhile boil the lids for 5 minutes.

Always heat your bottles to meet the temperature of your liquid to avoid cracking.

Safety Information and Warnings

Natural medicine is often considered safer than traditional medicine because it has no side effects. This is however slightly more complicated in that plants actually have many main effects (they may be good for coughs and colds but also be laxative too for example), therefore not all plants make suitable medicines for everyone. The ways they encourage hormones in the systems to alter can create damaging effects in some groups.

The main people to have concerns are:

1.	Diabetes sufferers

2.	Epilepsy patients

3.	Pregnant women

4.	Breast feeding women

5.	Suffers of rheumatism, arthritis and gout.

Diabetes
People with diabetes can safely use most plants with the exception of angelica. Plants which encourage the pancreas to work more effectively are dill and fennel and as such these are very helpful to suffers.

Epilepsy
Some plants have chemical constituents are which are neuro-toxic, this makes them dangerous not only to suffers of epilepsy but also some types of schizophrenia too.

Plants to avoid are: Rosemary, fennel, sage, eucalyptus, hyssop, camphor and spike lavender (Lavendula latifolia)

Pregnant Women
There are many actions which can make plants medicine dangerous in pregnancy. Most herbs and spices as well as fruits and vegetables can be eaten freely (except for penny royal mint and sage), but herbals and essential oils

should be avoided during the first 16 weeks and after that you should avoid Angelica, Black Pepper, Clove, Cypress, Eucalyptus, Ginger, Helichrysum, Marjoram, Myrrh, Nutmeg, Oregano, Peppermint, Roman Chamomile, Basil, Cassia, Cinnamon bark, Clary Sage, Lemongrass, Rosemary, Thyme, Vetiver, Wintergreen, White Fir.

Strong herbs and spices can be tasted in breast milk and so you may find they put the baby off feeding. Artichokes in particular are problematic. Meanwhile Carrot Seed Oil will enhance milk flow, geranium helps sooth engorged breasts and Marigold can heal cracked nipples all others should be used with care.

If baby does stop feeding avoid plant medicines for a day and see what happens.

Rheumatism, arthritis, gout, and also cystitis

This group of people should avoid foods which contain a constituent called Argenine found in asparagus and also spinach. More effective treatment might me to use juniper essential oil in their treatments.

Medicine From the Gardens

From the Veggie Patch

Beetroot
Rich in : Vitamins A, B, C, Magnesium, manganese, potassium & zinc.

Beetroot also contains an enzyme called Betane that regulates gastric juices and aids digestion. The leaves can also be cooked, are delicious in soups and are a tonic to the liver.

Artichoke
Rich in: Vitamins A B, C Folic Acid, Copper, Flouride, Manganese& Potassium

Artichokes are very healing to both the kidney and liver. They cleanse and nourish both organs and also aid with the absorption of fats in the system. It helps to lower levels of cholesterol.

Asparagus
Rich in: Vitamins A, B, C, Folic Acid, Copper, Fluoride, Manganese, Potassium, Asparagine

Asparagus is very diuretic and very low in calories. It aids intestinal health by inhibiting bacterial activity there. It is useful for breast feeding mothers as it promotes milk production.

The active ingredient asparagine is irritant to the following conditions: gout, rheumatism, arthritis, cystitis. See safety data.

Broccoli
Rich in: Vitamins A, C Folic Acid, E Calcium, Iron and Zinc

Believed to be an anti-cancer food, (along with cauliflower) broccoli is also a warrior against high blood pressure.

Cabbage
Rich in: A, B, C, K, E, potassium, sulphur and copper

Recommended as medicine to help the inflammation of the gut, cabbage water can help reduce stomach ulcers.

Used externally cabbage leaves ease the sting of eczema and burns. They reduce swelling from strains and sprains and are effective in fighting rheumatism, arthritis and gout.

Carrots
Rich in: Vitamin A, folic acid and iron+

The main uses for carrots are beauty related, cleansing and nourishing the skin. They also improve eczema and dermatitis. They are also very good aids to digestion and do, indeed, help improve vision.

Celery
Rich in: Vitamins A, B, C, Calcium, Magnesium, Manganese, Potassium

Celery alleviates digestive problems and also stimulates appetite. Relieving the build up of uric acid in the body it reduces the pain of rheumatism and arthritis. It breaks down kidney and bladder stones.

Courgette (Zuchinni)
Rich in: Vitamins A, B, C, Magnesium, phosphorous, potassium and zinc.

A very gentle vegetable, courgettes are recommended for sufferers of diabetes. They are mildly laxative and reduce inflammation in the kidneys and bladder. They are sedative too, and so are suggested as a part of a remedy strategy for insomnia.

Cucumber
Rich in: Vitamins A, B, C Iodine, Manganese and Sulphur

Cucumbers are full of water so are very good diuretics. They are anti-inflammatory (remember, on your eyes?) and help to dissolve uric acid. They hydrate and protect the skin.

Dandelion
Rich in: Vitamins A, B, C, Folic acid, calcium, iron, manganese, potassium and silica.

As previously stated, the use of dandelions for their diuretic and detoxifying properties is widespread and well recognised. Eating the leaves in salads is recommended for sufferers of poor liver function, gallbladder problems or kidney stones.

Lettuce
Rich in: Vitamin A, C, D, Folic Acid, E, Iron

This is a very ancient medicine. In the middle ages, lettuce was served at the beginning of a meal to stimulate appetite. It contains a constituent called lactucarium which is a powerful sedative. The perfect addition to a midnight snack, lettuce is recommended for treating insomnia.

The seeds of the lettuce are often overlooked but when made into a decoction makes a very healing remedy for asthma, bronchitis, spasmodic coughs and insomnia. This liquid can also be used externally to help conjunctivitis and acne.

Nettle
Rich in: Vitamins A, C, Carotene, Calcium, Iron, Magnesium, Potassium, Silica and Sulphur

Nettles make great additions to many recipes. Young leaves are tasty and eliminate uric acid from the system. They stimulate appetite and are wonderful to aid recuperation of poorly children. They combat infection. Better still, they reduce bleeding so amongst other conditions, menstrual problems are helped.

Peppers
Rich in: Vitamins A & C

Very beneficial for the heart, also use peppers to reduce diarrhoea, dyspepsia and gas.

Potatoes
Very alkaline, potatoes help to balance the acidity of psoriasis.

Pumpkin
Rich in: Folic acid, antioxidants and carotene

Pumpkins are a super food for sufferers of diabetes. They cleanse the bladder and kidneys of cystitis. Soaked in milk, their seeds aid insomnia. Soothe the flesh onto abscesses and wounds and to reduce inflammation.

Roasted seeds are a source of magnesium, phosphorous, zinc and potassium.

Spinach
Rich in: Vitamin C, Folic Acid, Iron, Zinc,

Rich in antioxidants, spinach stimulates pancreatic function. It is a powerful tonic and should be used to fight constipation. Overuse of spinach should be avoided as it can affect calcium absorption, leading to problems with gout etc (See safety.)

Tomato
Rich in: Vitamins A, B, C Folic acid, antioxidants

Tomatoes reduce inflammation of the bowel by reducing the bacterial activity there.

From the Flower Beds

Lavender
Lavender seeds are gorgeously relaxing and soothing. The essential oil makes a wonderful burn healer.

Rose
Full of estrogen, roses are gynaecological flowers. They reduce the effects of PMS and menopause. They also make beautiful skin foods; there is no better remedy for dry skin.

Geranium
The ultimate hormone balancer, it helps PMS, adolescence and menopause. Ultimately soothing, it is the perfect flower to lift away the problems of the day.

Camomile
Again, relaxing and soothing, especially for pain. Camomile is also digestive and anti-inflammatory.

Evening Primrose
The bright yellow flowers of this statuesque bush gladden your heart in summer. Its blossoms help to balance hormones and heal the sorest of skin conditions.

Violets
The genteel violet is extremely calming, especially to children. Very helpful for soothing very sensitive skins, it is also a powerful sedative helpful to insomnia.

Marigold
Opt for the calendula strain of marigold if you can, which is the gentlest and yet most powerful of all the skin healers

Ladies Mantle
The delicate ladies mantle has a way of overwhelming the flower borders sweeping everything out of its way. How appropriate, as it is the very best treatment for Premenstrual Syndrome. (I wonder if that is how it gained its name.)

Comfrey

Our forbearers called this Knit bone. It heals broken bones and wounds very quickly.

From the Herb Garden

Basil
Basil has digestive properties which help abdominal cramps and colic. Its best qualities though, are for helping the nervous system. Anxiety, insomnia, and mental fatigue are all improved, and should be the first herb you pick to reduce a migraine.

Bay
This is the perfect herb to use to get rid of "that bloated feeling" Whether it is from poor diet or a familiar monthly visit, bay is a wonderful help.

Borage
Another excellent skin tonic, borage helps dry scaly conditions such as eczema and psoriasis. It is also very good for calming the "madness" of menopause, from hot flashes to mood swings.

It is a useful find for anyone with either blood issues or diabetes. It regulates blood sugar, reduces blood pressure and also naturally thins the blood.

Coriander (Cilantro)
Digestive as you might imagine, but coriander is also antibiotic too. Sprinkle it, raw, onto soups, curries and salads to help get rid of a cold.

Marjoram
Marjoram is powerful tonic to the central nervous system. Use it in small amounts to help anxiety and insomnia.

Mint
As you would imagine, mint is digestive and helps to reduce nausea and vomiting. It helps to reduce palpitations and is great for clearing the mind. It is very cooling and refreshing.

The leaves are also very helpful for clearing the airways of bronchitis and asthma.

Before using in pregnancy please review the **Safety Data** *before using this herb.*

Oregano
A very powerful antibiotic, this is helpful to clear out bugs and germs.

Parsley
Parsley is a very useful herb. The leaves are best eaten raw and will help with flatulence, but also stimulate appetite and liver function. It is also a very good anti-aging ingredient the leaves are rubbed into the skin as part of a facial.

Rosemary
A very good herb for digestion but its primary functions are to help reduce nerve pain, whether associated with rheumatism, sciatica or neuralgia.

For suffers of epilepsy, please review the **Safety Data** *before using this herb.*

Tarragon
A general all round stimulant, tarragon is the ultimate tonic. Use it at the beginning of winter to boost your immune system before the onslaught of colds and other nastiness. It helps muscular aches and pains and also reduces menstrual pains.

For suffers of epilepsy, please review the **Safety Data** *before using this herb.*

Thyme
There is a huge diversity in the different subspecies of thyme. Unlike mints whose properties change between species, thyme tends to have very similar uses right across the family.

These are: intestinal worms and parasites, improves circulation, reduces bronchitis and coughs.

Lemon Balm
The beautiful fresh Melissa plant is anti-allergenic. It helps to reduce seizures and fitting. It is also now recommended in essential oil form to help cognition in sufferers of epilepsy. It is uplifting to the spirits; pure sunshine!

Dill
A very good digestive, this is the plant which is used in Gripe Water to sooth babies' colic.

From the Orchard

Poetic license, I wish my orchard looked like this list. Clearly these are spread from across the globe.

Apricot
Rich in: Vitamins A, B, C Iron, magnesium and Manganese

These are very balancing to the nervous system and so are great for anxiety. How about stuffing a few into school lunch boxes the week before exams? They are also very good for fatigue and are especially recommended for pregnant ladies. They are a tonic for the blood and help anaemia, as well as the elderly and those who are convalescing.

Blackberry
Rich in: Vitamins A, B, C Calcium, Iron and Phosphorous

If you, like me, have brambles which refuse to be tamed, you will be pleased to hear they do have their uses. The leaves are used to help sore throats. A syrup made from the fruit reduces diarrhoea, and is a great tonic for sickly children.

Blackcurrant
Rich in: Vitamin C

We all recognise this drink from our youth I am sure. It speeds recuperation after illness and aids in remineralisation of bones after breakages and fractures.

Dates
Rich in: Vitamins A, B, D Calcium, Magnesium and Potassium

Research shows that dates may be instrumental in preventing cancer. They improve circulation and are a tonic for anaemia. In North African traditional medicine the boiled and powdered stones (or pits) are used to treat Tuberculosis. Here, the fruit is recommended for respiratory problems too.

Figs
Rich in: Vitamins A, B, C, Folic Acid, Calcium, Copper, Iron, Potassium and Zinc

Constipation, I am sure you know. They are also excellent help for sore throats and bronchitis.

Guava
Rich in: Vitamin C, Potassium, Sulphur.

Very astringent, guavas are fabulous skin cleansers. They are also good for digestion but beware of unripe fruits which can be harmful to people with intestinal problems.

Lemon
Rich in: A, B, C, Potassium, Phosphorous and Copper

The herbal doctor's best friend, lemon oozes vitamin C. It is astringent and cleansing as well as being antiseptic. For anyone suffering from circulatory problems, lemon is a boon as it strengthens the arterial walls allowing the blood to pump more vitally.

Mandarin
See orange, however mandarin is also a tonic for adrenal system which becomes exhausted when we are stressed.

Mango
Rich in: Vitamins A, B, C Phosphorous and Sulphur

The mango's main effect is on contractions. Useful in pregnancy and labour, certainly, however most effective is the aid it gives to ulcerative colitis and Irritable Bowel Syndrome.

Melon
Rich in: Vitamins A, B, C

Cooling and refreshing, melon is also anti-inflammatory. Melon can be used to treat mild burns (for more severe burns opt for lavender) and also sunburn.

Melons are also laxative and because of their high juice content are diuretic too.

Orange
Rich in: Vitamins B, C, copper, calcium and phosphorous

Stimulate the immune system, liver and also appetite.

Papaya
Rich in: Vitamins A, B, C and potassium

Reduces fever.

Plum
Rich in: Calcium, iron, magnesium

Laxative, but also reduce cholesterol in the blood.

Prune
See plums.

Raspberry
Rich in: Vitamin A, B, C, Iron, Magnesium and potassium

Raspberries help to reduce frequent urination. A tea made from raspberry leaves will help to strengthen contractions in labour. Do not drink until after the 35th week of pregnancy.

Healing Recipes

What follows is a selection of ideas of how to implement the fore mentioned ingredients into your daily life.

There is only one hard set rule and that is this: do not use plant medicine to replace a doctor's advice. There is a good reason they train for many more years than herbalists and aroma-therapists; please keep taking your prescribed drugs and talk to your doctor about the remedies in this book. In many parts of the world you will find practitioners are more open to natural medicine than you might think.

Other than that one rule, break free, experiment, research and find your own healing medium. For some the garden provides everything they need, others choose to rely on extracts and even crystals.

So, without further ado....lets create some medicine!

Elizabeth Fellow

The Respiratory System

Recipes for Colds

Comforting Nettle Soup
Pick fresh young leaves from the top of the plant. Try to source them away from roads and polluted areas.

500g (18 oz) Potatoes

300g (10oz) Nettle leaves and stems

75ml (3 oz) Olive Oil

2 Tbs finely chopped parsley

Peel and chop the potatoes. Cover with cold water, bring to the boil and simmer for 20 mins or until cooked.

Add the nettle tops and continue to cook for another 5- 8 mins

Season with salt and pepper.

Liquidise in a food processor.

Stir in the olive oil.

Garnish with the parsley and some golden croutons.

Papaya Pick Me Up

2 ripe papayas

2 chopped bananas

Juice of 2 limes

Lime zest

3 tbsp of Greek yogurt

600ml (21 fl oz) apple juice

Dice the flesh of the papayas and chopped bananas into a food processor. Add the juices, zest and yogurt and process until smooth.

Lemon and Ginger Shoo Flu
1 cm Nub of fresh ginger, grated or finely chopped

1 Lemon

1 tbsp of honey

500 ml (18 fl oz) boiling water

Place the ginger into a heavy bottomed saucepan.

Grate the zest from the lemon and place into the pan.

Squeeze out all of the juice and add to the mixture.

Cover with boiling water. Bring back to the boil and simmer gently for 8 minutes.

Drink hot.

Recipes for Sore Throats

Feel Better Fig Infused Apple Juice

3 Figs – Finely chopped

25 g (1 oz) Camomile Flowers (or a camomile tea bag)

250 ml (9 fl oz) Apple Juice

2 tsp honey

Place the figs and camomile into a small saucepan and add the honey.

Add the apple juice and heat gently for 8 minutes. Do not allow to boil.

Drink Warm.

Baked Papaya and Ginger Soothing Hug

2 papayas halved and seeded

60g (2 oz) unsalted butter

5 chunks of preserved stem ginger

Juice and zest of a lime

1 tbs of the syrup from the ginger jar

Preheat oven to 180 Degrees Celcius / 350 Degrees Fahrenheit/ Gas Mark 4

Mash together the ginger, syrup and lime.

Place the papayas in an ovenproof dish

Coat thoroughly with the ginger-lime mix

Bake in for 20 mins, turning regularly.

Serve with a drizzle of honey.

Giggle Again Guava Shake

When all else fails numb your throat with this shake laden with Vitamin C and healing energies.

100g (4 oz) strawberries (quartered)

50 g (2 oz) guava

150g (6 oz) strawberry yogurt

1 frozen banana

5 ice cubes

Whizz all of the ingredients together in the food processor. Drink cold

Cheating Healer's Sore Throat Gargle

75 ml (3fl oz) Glass of warm water

½ Aspirin

2 drops of Tea Tree oil

1 drop Lavender oil

Dissolve the aspirin into the water and add the essential oils.

Gargle the heinous tasting brew to relieve the soreness and attack the germs with antibiotic oils. <u>Do NOT swallow</u>.

Booster Blackberry Syrup

1 kg (35 oz) Blackberries

1 kg (35 oz) Sugar

150 ml (5 fl oz) water

Bring all of the ingredients to the boil. Simmer for 10 minutes. Pour into a sterilised bottle. Seal tightly and refrigerate.

Dosage: 1 tsp 150 ml water.

For *extra-comfort-and-my-bed-please* kind of days add to warm water or even better…warmed apple juice.

For Chest Infections, Bronchitis & Asthma

Purifying Parsley & Nettle Inhalation
100g (4 oz) parsley, dried or fresh, finely chopped

100g (4 oz) nettles

Boiling Water

See: How to make inhalants

The Skeleton and Skin

For Orthopaedic Injury

Comfrey Poultice
6 large comfrey leaves

50 ml (2 fl oz) water

100ml (4 oz) Gram Flour (plain flour will work just as well if you can't find gram)

Optional: To improve the healing even further add 100g (4 oz) each of courgette (zucchini) and pumpkin flesh.

Place the leaves (plus the courgette and pumpkin if used) with water in a blender to make a pulp. Stir in the flour to make a more manageable paste.

Smear onto gauze and apply to the wound.

Secure into place with a bandage and if desired, cling film to protect from leakage.

Leave on for 8 hours.

Repeat as often as necessary. Residue mixture can be kept for up to 3 days if covered and stored in the refrigerator.

Recipes to Aid in Skin Healing

Summer Garden Skin Delight
Collect marigold, evening primrose, borage, and rose petals from the garden on an early summer's morning.

Place in a jar. Cover with vegetable oil. Place on the windowsill to infuse for 1 month.

Use this maceration as a skin healing oil.

Borage Tea
25 g Leaves and flowers

Place into a teapot and cover with boiling water.

Allow to infuse for 5 minutes.

Drink warm to boost the body's skin healing abilities.

Borage Poultice for Troublesome Skin (Ideal for Eczema and Psoriasis)
50g (2 oz) Borage leaves and flowers finely chopped

1 Tbs of Summer Garden Skin Delight or Almond Oil

One Packet of dried Yeast

Very strong borage tea infusion left to steep for 25 minutes

Mix together the ingredients and smear onto the skin. Leave on for 10 minutes. Rinse away, past dry and apply moisturiser.

Verrucaes (Plantar's Warts)

The old ones recommend using dandelion juice on the area. A more effective treatment is to apply undiluted lemon and tea tree essential oils onto the wart using cotton swabs. Be careful not to get lemon oil on unaffected skin as it is irritant.

Athletes Foot

Rub a couple of drops of tea tree oil on the affected parts of the feet. Put a couple of drops into the final rinse in the washing machine to completely eradicate the fungal infection spores from any socks the sufferer has been wearing.

Hair Glosses

To make your hair gleam in the sunshine use herbal infusions as your final hair rinse.

For dark hair

5 large sprigs of rosemary, lightly chopped

500 ml (18 fl oz) of boiling water

1 tsp cider vinegar

For lighter hair and redheads

25g (1 oz) Camomile Flowers

Juice of half a lemon (*Redheads may want to omit the lemon juice as it helps the sun to lighten the tone of the hair using a slightly bleaching effect.*)

500 ml (18 fl oz) boiling water

1 tsp Cider Vinegar

Bring the mix to the boil and then simmer for 20 minutes.

Refrigerate for 30 minutes before using.

Use cold.

The Genito- Urinary System

Menstrual Pains and PMS

Ladies Mantle Secret Soak
Pick lavender seeds, camomile and ladies mantle

Cut out a circle of muslin 8 inches in diameter

Place the flowers into the middle.

Bunch the fabric around the flowers and fasten with a piece of ribbon.

Float the sachet in your warm bath, and allow the water to infuse with the healing essential oils.

Reuse for two days after then dispose of the sachet.

Premenstrual Promise

Collect Rose petals, ladies mantle, lavender seeds, jasmine blossoms and Camomile flowers from the garden on an early summer's morning. Create a maceration from the blooms and let steep for 1 month.

Gently smooth over the abdomen and lower back in problem weeks.

Also make a deliciously, luxurious massage oil.

Menopausal Symptoms
See Borage Tea

Make a maceration of Rose, Geranium and Camomile Flowers. Massage over the uterus and lower back daily.

Cystitis (Bladder Infection)

Come on; Stop Laughing At Me Pumpkin Detox!

Sadly, you are going to have to let someone witness "the crazy" with this one as I have found it virtually impossible to apply yourself!

250 g (9 oz) Cooked Pumpkin pulp

50ml (2 fl oz) warm water

50g (2 oz) Gram Flour

4 drops tea tree oil

Cover your bed with a towel before you lie down.

Mix the ingredients together to make a thick paste. Lie down and ask a friend to smear the mix over your lower back, in the region of the kidneys.

Lay a warm towel over you to keep warm and leave on for 20 minutes.

Rise away with warm water.

Drink Lemon and Ginger Shoo Flu

Don't forget the traditional favourite, bottles and bottles of cranberry juice.

The Digestive and Excretory System

Indigestion

Make an infusion from peppermint leaves and steep for 5 minutes.

Drink warm or cold.

Constipation

8 fresh figs, quartered

100 ml (4 oz) boiling water

100 g (4 oz) sugar

Juice of 1 lemon

Optional: For extra drive and oomph add 18 g (3/4 oz) Senna Pods

Follow the instructions for syrups, this time leaving the mix to simmer for 25 minutes. Strain the contents before adding to a sterilised bottle.

Take one tsp before bed to allow the bowels plenty of time to process.

Nature's Medicine

Just a Regular Breakfast

3 Figs

100g (4 oz) Ricotta Cheese

2tbs Greek Honey

Arrange the cheese and figs on a plate, drizzle with honey.

This'll Get Ya Moving Fruit Salad!

Plums, Figs, Melons

'Nuff said!

Diarrhoea

Crème de Cassis or Blackcurrant Syrup

500g (18 oz) Blackcurrants

500g (18 oz) Sugar

Take a large

jar and thinly layer, fruit, sugar, fruit sugar all the way up the jar.

Leave to rest in a dark place for 6 months

Strain into sterilized jars.

This syrup will keep indefinitely if stored out of light.

Take as and when desired. Dilute with water.

For an extra special treat add to white wine for a bit of after dinner luxury.

Ginger is a wonderful ingredient for any condition where the body is struggling to cope with excess moisture. Therefore, treat yourself to a warm cup of Lemon and Ginger Shoo Flu

Colitis and IBS

Asparagus Syrup
200ml (7fl oz) of asparagus juice (extract using a juicer)

400g (14 oz) sugar

See: How to make syrups

Boil for 15 minutes until thickened.

Store in sterilized jars

Digestive Delight Vegetable Tincture

This tincture allows you to have the healing effects of the vegetables without the impact of all the fibre on the gut.

1 Raw Beetroot,

3 Carrot,

2 sticks Celery,

1 Red Pepper,

3 medium tomatoes

250ml (9 fl oz) Vodka

Process the vegetables in a food processor. Add to the alcohol. Follow How to make tinctures. Take 30 drops on 75 ml (2.5 oz.) water morning and evening

Nausea
Enjoy an infusion of peppermint Tea

Or how about a taste of the orient with:

Ginger and Mandarin Infusion
1cm nub of ginger roughly chopped

300ml (10 fl oz) boiling water

Juice of a mandarin

1tsp honey

Bring the water to the boil and add the ginger. Simmer for 5 minutes. Add to juice of the orange and honey and cook for 2 more minutes.

Allow to cool slightly before drinking.

The Circulatory System

Haemorrhoids
Make a cold compress with a flannel or tissue. Use 5 drops of geranium essential oil on the pad. Apply to the affected part after each bowel movement

Macerations made with geraniums also make a good oil to smooth around the anus for healing between bowel movements.

Thin Blood
Dried apricots, apricot muesli, baked apricots....no secrets here, just use your imagination.

Improve Clotting
I know of no plant medicine that will improve the clotting efficiency of the blood, but calcium supplements are extremely effective.

To Reduce High Blood Pressure
Broccoli, cauliflower should feature regularly on your plate. Also try making:

Rosemary Tincture
25g (1oz) Dried rosemary

150ml (6 fl oz) Vodka

See How to make tinctures.

Dosage: 30 drops in 75 ml water.

No suitable for those with epilepsy

The Muscular System & Aches and Pains

Rheumatism, Arthritis and Gout

Goodbye Aches and Pains Cabbage, Carrot and Blueberry Juice

2 Parts Fresh Cabbage Juice

2 parts Fresh Carrot Juice

1 Part Blue Berry Juice

Extract each juice individually using a juicer, then combine and drink.

Creaking Cabbage and Courgette Poultice

Gently boil 4 cabbage leaves and a sliced courgette (zucchini) for 5 minutes.

Strain and squeeze out excess juice.

Lay the pulp onto a gauze.

Bandage over the affected part and leave for 20 minutes.

Muscular Pain
Draw a warm bath and add 5 drops each of lavender and geranium oils.

Oohs and Aahs Gentle Rub
Make a maceration of

5 sprigs of fresh rosemary leaves,

10 sprigs of basil leaves and stalks

2 tbs lavender flowers

1 tbs geranium flower heads

Rub into weary and tired muscles.

The Lymphatic System

Water Retention

Diminish You, Dandelion Tea

Look on any natural weight loss packet and you will find dandelion on the label. It truly is a wonder herb! For tea, use only leaves although petals and roots are also safe and tasty to eat.

Use 10 big, juicy, fresh green leaves and pour over with hot water.

Steep for 5 minutes.

Sweeten with honey.

Flush Out Fennel Seed Decoction

Fennel tea is wonderful for reducing bloating but here's just a bit of variety for you.

25g (1 oz) Fennel Seeds

300ml (10 fl oz) boiling water

Follow How to make Decoctions and drink warm.

Use the same recipe in two bases. Make a massage oil and then also a clay to be smeared over the buttocks and legs very much like you would a face mask.

The mask is hilarious fun but messy. Grab a girlfriend for a spa evening so you can help each other apply the treatments. Ensure you cover surfaces with some old towels and wash them straight afterwards.

For Massage Oil

2 Drops Grapefruit Essential oil

2 Drops Fennel Essential oil

2 Drops Rosemary Essential Oil

100 ml (4 fl oz) vegetable oil

For Clay Mask

25g (1 oz) packet of green or red clay (available from health food shops) and 10ml (1/2 fl oz) vegetable oil.

Smear on the clay then cover with a cling film wrap.

Leave on for 20 minutes before showering away.

Follow with a soothing massage with the cellulite massage oil.

The Nervous System and Emotions

Headaches and Migraine

Make a maceration of lavender, camomile, basil, rosemary from your garden. Massage onto the back of the neck when you feel a headache coming on and also on the temples.

Peppermint tea is also often helpful.

You could also try:

Camomile Tea

25g (1 oz) Camomile Flower Heads

300 ml (10 fl oz) of boiling water

Steep for 5 -10 minutes.

Sweeten with honey and drink warm.

Insomnia

Lettuce on your sandwiches, courgettes (zucchini) on your plate and of course not forgetting a great big slice of pumpkin pie! But how about we try something slightly more unusual?

Aunt Violet's Sleepy Syrup

About 6 handfuls of sweet violet flowers

300ml (10 fl oz) water

600g (21 oz) sugar

Remove all of the greenery from the flowers, keeping only those dreamy purple blooms.

Place them into a ceramic bowl and set it on top of a saucepan to make a bain-marie.

Boil water in the pan below to heat the bowl then pour the 300ml of water over the flowers.

Leave them to steep overnight.

Next day, strain the violet juice off and return to the bain marie.

Reheat to boiling temperature and add the sugar.

Stirring often let the syrup thicken for about 15 minutes.

Store in sterilized jars.

Use as a medicine for insomnia by diluting in water or use neat on ice creams and cakes.

Restful Sleep Massage Oil
100 mls (4 fl oz) Vegetable oil

3 drops Lavender oil

1 drop Marjoram oil

Use daily to aid sleep.

And lastly, use your imagination to soothe your own emotions or ease others in your home. Here are a few combinations which you might like to use.

Relaxation

Geranium, lavender, camomile

Anger

Rose, geranium

Nerves

Rosemary, Apricots, mandarin

Romance

Rose, jasmine.

Conclusion

So, if you have found your way to this last page, I'll take it as a compliment! I hope you have enjoyed this little foraging foray. Who knows perhaps our paths will one day cross in some mossy woodland both grasping for the same berries!

Plant medicine is a fascinating subject, not least because of the fact every day we learn something new; a new recipe, often a new restricting legislation or even an unheard of disease which attacks our world, this is how nature creates and destroys.

So now you carry with you not only wisdom, but also a responsibility to protect and preserve this precious kingdom. Please, grow some treasures yourself. Whether it be a pot of basil on the windowsill or even those wretched stinging nettles at the bottom of garden, make sure you give a little bit back.

In terms of gratitude, I would like to say my own thank you to a few authors who have added a great deal to the research of this book. Pierre Jean Cousin and his wonderful book Food is Medicine, Carol Vorderman and her iconic 28 day Detox, Dr Jean Valnet- Practical Aromatherapy, Jill Bruce – The Garden of Eden and Fiona Summers –Introduction to Aromatherapy. These people's works have shaped my own views and the love I have for plants to pass on to future generations.

I wonder what medicine will look like to our grandchildren. Will antibiotics have any strength by then and will AIDs have been cured? Will their drugs be synthetically engineered or might they have seeded naturally by the compost heap?

Who knows, perhaps we will live long enough to see. I hope so.

Be creative, be healthy but most of all dear reader use your plants to have a happy and peaceful live.

I wish you well.

Elizabeth Fellow

Please leave a review and let us know what you liked about this book by going to

https://www.amazon.com/gp/css/order-history

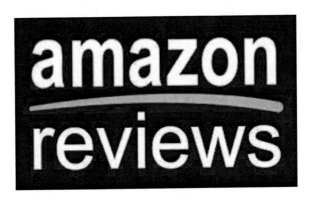

then clicking on Orders.

CPSIA information can be obtained at www.ICGtesting.com
Printed in the USA
LVOW10s1954071214

417651LV00029B/893/P